The Postpartum Survival Guide

The Postpartum Survival Guide

Suzanne Byrd

CONTENTS

- 2　Recognizing the Symptoms　6
- 3　The Diagnosis Process　11
- 4　Treatment Options Overview　16
- 5　Medication and PND　21
- 6　Psychotherapy Approaches　26
- 7　Impact on Family Dynamics　32
- 8　Societal Stigma and Mental Health　37
- 9　Building a Support Network　42
- 10　Self-Care Strategies for New Mothers　47
- 11　Preventing Postnatal Depression　53
- 12　Moving Forward: Recovery and Hope　58

Copyright © 2025 by Suzanne Byrd
All rights reserved. No part of this book may be reproduced in any manner whatsoever without written permission except in the case of brief quotations embodied in critical articles and reviews.
First Printing, 2025

Introduction to Postnatal Depression

Chapter 1: Introduction to Postnatal Depression

Introduction to Postnatal Depression

The birth of a child is often portrayed as one of life's most joyous occasions, a moment filled with celebration and love. Yet for many new mothers, the weeks and months following delivery can be marked by overwhelming sadness, exhaustion, and a profound sense of isolation. This is the reality of Postnatal Depression (PND), a serious mental health condition that affects countless women worldwide. Despite its prevalence, PND remains shrouded in silence, often dismissed as mere "baby blues" or a temporary phase. This chapter serves as a vital introduction to PND, offering clarity on what it is, why it happens, and how to recognize its signs. By shedding light on this often-misunderstood condition, we aim to empower women to seek the help they deserve and break the stigma that prevents so many from speaking up.

What is Postnatal Depression?

Postnatal Depression is a clinical condition that goes far beyond the fleeting mood swings commonly referred to as the "baby blues." While the baby blues—characterized by mild sadness, irritability, and fatigue—typically resolve within two weeks of childbirth, PND is more severe and persistent. It can emerge anytime within the first year after delivery and often lingers without proper intervention.

The symptoms of PND are multifaceted, affecting emotional, physical, and psychological well-being. Emotionally, mothers may experience unrelenting sadness, hopelessness, or numbness, even in moments that "should" bring happiness. Physically, they might struggle with extreme fatigue, changes in appetite, or unexplained aches and pains. Psychologically, PND can manifest as intrusive thoughts, guilt over perceived inadequacy as a mother, or even difficulty bonding with the baby.

Biologically, PND is linked to dramatic hormonal shifts after childbirth, particularly the rapid drop in estrogen and progesterone. These changes can disrupt brain chemistry, exacerbating vulnerability to depression. However, PND is not solely a hormonal issue—it is influenced by a complex interplay of genetic predisposition, personal history of mental health struggles, lack of social support, and the immense pressures of new motherhood. Recognizing PND as a legitimate medical condition is the first step toward effective treatment and recovery.

Prevalence and Underreporting

Research indicates that approximately 1 in 7 women experience Postnatal Depression, making it one of the most common complications of childbirth. Yet, despite its prevalence, PND is significantly underreported. Many mothers suffer in silence, fearing judgment or believing their struggles are a personal failing rather than a treatable condition.

Societal stigma plays a major role in this underreporting. The idealized image of the "perfect mother" who effortlessly embraces her new role leaves little room for vulnerability. Women may worry about being labeled as "ungrateful" or "unfit" if they admit to struggling. Cultural barriers further compound the issue; in some communities, mental health discussions are taboo, leaving mothers without the language or support to express their pain.

Consider the case of Sarah, a first-time mother who dismissed her exhaustion and tearfulness as normal adjustments. It wasn't until her partner noticed her withdrawing from family life that she sought help. Stories like Sarah's are far too common, highlighting the urgent need for greater awareness and open dialogue.

The Importance of Awareness

Awareness is a powerful tool in combating PND. When mothers, families, and healthcare providers understand the signs and risks, early intervention becomes possible. Education can dismantle myths—such as the belief that PND is a sign of weakness—and replace them with empathy and actionable support.

For new mothers, awareness begins with self-compassion. Understanding that PND is not a choice or a character flaw, but a medical condition, can alleviate guilt and encourage seeking help. Families and friends play a crucial role by educating themselves on PND, offering nonjudgmental support, and recognizing when professional intervention may be needed.

Resources such as postpartum support groups, mental health hotlines, and online communities can provide invaluable guidance. Organizations like Postpartum Support International offer evidence-based information and connections to local specialists. By prioritizing awareness, we create a safety net for mothers who might otherwise suffer alone.

Recognizing the Signs

Early recognition of PND symptoms can dramatically improve outcomes. While every mother's experience is unique, common signs include:

- Persistent sadness or emptiness that lasts most of the day
- Loss of interest in activities once enjoyed
- Difficulty bonding with the baby or feeling emotionally detached
- Overwhelming fatigue, even after adequate rest
- Changes in appetite—either significant weight loss or gain
- Intense irritability, anxiety, or anger
- Feelings of worthlessness or excessive guilt
- Thoughts of self-harm or harming the baby (in severe cases)

It's important to note that PND doesn't always look like classic depression. Some mothers may appear functional on the outside while battling inner turmoil. If you or someone you know exhibits these symptoms for more than two weeks, it's crucial to consult a healthcare provider. Keeping a journal of mood changes and symptoms can help during medical evaluations.

Breaking the Stigma

The stigma surrounding PND is one of the biggest barriers to treatment. Too often, mothers are told to "snap out of it" or "cherish this precious time," invalidating their pain. Breaking this stigma requires collective effort—starting with honest conversations.

Public figures like actress Chrissy Teigen and singer Adele have bravely shared their PND experiences, helping to normalize the condition. Their openness reminds us that PND does not discriminate; it can affect anyone, regardless of background or circumstance.

On a personal level, we can combat stigma by:

- Speaking openly about mental health without shame
- Challenging harmful stereotypes about motherhood
- Encouraging healthcare providers to screen for PND routinely
- Offering practical support to new mothers, such as meal deliveries or childcare

Creating a culture where mothers feel safe to ask for help is not just beneficial—it's lifesaving.

Conclusion

Postnatal Depression is a profound and often misunderstood challenge, but it is not insurmountable. By understanding its nature, recognizing its signs, and fostering a supportive environment, we can transform the narrative around PND from one of shame to one of hope. If you're reading this and see yourself in these words, know that you are not alone, and help is available. If you're a partner, friend, or family member, your awareness and compassion can make all the difference. Together, we can ensure that no mother has to face Postnatal Depression in silence.

The journey through PND begins with knowledge—and this chapter is your first step. In the following pages, we'll explore practical strategies for coping, healing, and reclaiming joy in motherhood.

Recognizing the Symptoms

Chapter 2: Recognizing the Symptoms

The arrival of a new baby is often portrayed as a time of joy and fulfillment, yet for many women, the postpartum period can be overshadowed by overwhelming emotions, exhaustion, and a sense of disconnect. Postnatal depression (PND) affects approximately 1 in 7 women, yet it remains widely misunderstood and frequently dismissed as mere "baby blues." Recognizing the symptoms of PND is the first critical step toward seeking help and reclaiming emotional well-being. This chapter will guide you through the emotional, physical, and behavioral signs of PND, clarify when these symptoms typically emerge, and empower you to break through the stigma that often prevents women from seeking the support they deserve.

Emotional Symptoms: More Than Just 'Baby Blues'

The emotional toll of postnatal depression extends far beyond the fleeting mood swings commonly associated with the "baby blues." While it's normal to feel tearful or overwhelmed in the first two weeks after childbirth due to hormonal fluctuations and sleep deprivation, PND is characterized by persistent and intense emotional distress.

Women with PND often describe a deep, unshakable sadness that lingers for weeks or months. Feelings of hopelessness, worthlessness, or guilt—particularly about not being a "good enough" mother—are common. Irritability and anger may surface unexpectedly, even toward loved ones or the baby, which can further fuel guilt and shame. Anxiety is another hallmark symptom, manifesting as excessive worry about the baby's health, irrational fears of harm, or a paralyzing sense of dread about the future.

Perhaps one of the most painful aspects of PND is the sense of detachment from the baby. Some women report feeling numb or indifferent, as if they're going through the motions of caregiving without the expected emotional bond. This detachment can be deeply distressing, compounding feelings of failure.

Consider the story of Maria, a first-time mother who assumed her exhaustion and tearfulness were normal. But when her sadness persisted beyond the first month, accompanied by intrusive thoughts about her baby's safety, she realized something was wrong. With support, Maria learned these were classic signs of PND—not a personal failing.

Physical Symptoms: The Body's Silent Alarm

Postnatal depression doesn't just affect the mind; it takes a tangible toll on the body. Unfortunately, many women dismiss these physical symptoms as inevitable side effects of new motherhood, delaying diagnosis and treatment.

Chronic fatigue is one of the most common yet overlooked signs. While sleep deprivation is expected with a newborn, PND-related exhaustion feels unrelenting, as if no amount of rest can replenish energy levels. Changes in appetite—either loss of interest in food or compulsive eating—are also red flags. Some women experience unexplained aches and pains, headaches, or digestive issues, which may be misattributed to postpartum recovery.

Sleep disturbances are particularly insidious. Even when the baby sleeps, women with PND may struggle with insomnia or wake frequently due to anxiety. Conversely, some find themselves sleeping excessively yet never feeling rested.

Take the example of Jessica, who assumed her constant fatigue and migraines were just part of adjusting to motherhood. It wasn't until her doctor connected these symptoms to her emotional state that she recognized they were part of a larger issue. Paying attention to these physical cues can be a vital step in identifying PND.

Behavioral Changes: Recognizing Patterns

Behavioral shifts often serve as outward indicators of internal struggles. Women with PND may withdraw from social interactions, canceling plans with friends or avoiding family gatherings. Activities that once brought joy—reading, exercising, or creative hobbies—may suddenly feel meaningless.

Difficulty concentrating or making decisions is another telltale sign. Simple tasks like grocery shopping or responding to emails can feel overwhelming. Some women describe a mental fog, as if their thoughts are moving through molasses. Neglect of self-care, such as skipping showers or wearing the same clothes for days, can also signal PND.

These behavioral changes can strain relationships. Partners may feel confused or hurt by the withdrawal, while friends might misinterpret the lack of engagement as disinterest. In reality, these patterns reflect the isolating grip of PND.

Sarah's story illustrates this well. An outgoing woman before childbirth, she began declining invitations and stopped texting friends. Her husband grew concerned when she spent hours staring blankly at the TV. Only after a candid conversation did they realize these behaviors were symptoms of PND, not a new personality trait.

When Do Symptoms Appear? Timing Matters

Understanding the timeline of PND is crucial for early intervention. While some women experience symptoms within the first few weeks postpartum, others may not notice changes until months later.

Early-onset PND typically emerges within the first four weeks after delivery. Hormonal shifts, physical recovery, and the abrupt transition to motherhood can trigger overwhelming emotions. Late-onset PND, which can develop up to a year postpartum, is often linked to prolonged stress, lack of support, or unmet expectations about motherhood.

External factors—such as financial strain, relationship difficulties, or a traumatic birth experience—can also influence when symptoms surface. Sleep deprivation, a near-universal challenge for new mothers, exacerbates emotional vulnerability, making it harder to cope.

Monitoring your mental health during this period is essential. If low moods, anxiety, or physical symptoms persist beyond two weeks or intensify over time, it's important to seek professional guidance.

Breaking the Stigma: Seeking Help Without Shame

Despite its prevalence, postnatal depression is still shrouded in stigma. Many women fear being labeled as "ungrateful" or "weak" if they admit to struggling. This silence only deepens isolation and delays recovery.

It's time to reframe the narrative: Seeking help is an act of courage, not failure. PND is a medical condition, not a character flaw. Just as you would seek treatment for a physical ailment, your mental health deserves the same care.

Start by confiding in someone you trust—a partner, friend, or healthcare provider. Support groups, both in-person and online, can provide validation and practical advice from women who've walked this path. Therapy, medication, or a combination of both are proven, effective treatments.

Remember Maria, Jessica, and Sarah? Each of them found healing by reaching out. You can too.

Conclusion: A Path Forward

Recognizing the symptoms of postnatal depression is the first step toward reclaiming your well-being. Whether you're grappling with emotional turmoil, physical exhaustion, or behavioral changes, know that these experiences are not your fault—and they are not permanent. By understanding the signs and rejecting the stigma, you empower yourself to seek the support you deserve.

Postnatal depression is treatable. With awareness, compassion, and timely intervention, you can navigate this challenging chapter and emerge stronger. You are not alone, and help is within reach. The journey to healing begins with a single, brave step: acknowledging that you matter, just as much as your baby does.

3

The Diagnosis Process

Chapter 3: The Diagnosis Process

The journey through motherhood is often painted in hues of joy and fulfillment, but for many women, the postpartum period can be overshadowed by an unexpected and overwhelming emotional struggle. Postnatal depression (PND) affects approximately one in seven women, yet it remains widely misunderstood and frequently underdiagnosed. Recognizing and diagnosing PND is a critical step toward recovery, yet the process is fraught with challenges—ranging from societal stigma to the subtlety of symptoms that mimic typical postpartum adjustments. This chapter explores the diagnosis process in depth, shedding light on the role of healthcare providers, the tools used to identify PND, and the barriers that often delay or obscure an accurate diagnosis. By understanding these elements, women and their support networks can take proactive steps toward seeking the help they deserve.

The Role of Healthcare Providers

Healthcare providers serve as the first line of defense in identifying postnatal depression. From obstetricians and midwives to general practitioners and pediatricians, these professionals are uniquely positioned to recognize early warning signs. However, the responsibility does not rest solely on their shoulders. Open communication between mothers and their healthcare teams is paramount.

Postpartum check-ups are often focused on physical recovery, but mental health assessments should be an integral part of these visits. Many women hesitate to voice their emotional struggles, fearing they will be dismissed as "normal" postpartum blues or, worse, judged as inadequate mothers. To bridge this gap, healthcare providers must create a safe, non-judgmental space where women feel comfortable sharing their experiences.

For mothers preparing for these appointments, it can be helpful to jot down symptoms beforehand, noting their frequency and intensity. Questions like, "Are my feelings interfering with daily life?" or "Have I lost interest in activities I once enjoyed?" can guide the conversation. Additionally, bringing a trusted partner or friend to the appointment can provide emotional support and help articulate concerns.

Common Diagnostic Tools

Accurate diagnosis of postnatal depression relies on validated screening tools designed to distinguish between typical postpartum adjustments and clinically significant depression. The most widely used instrument is the Edinburgh Postnatal Depression Scale (EPDS), a 10-question self-report questionnaire that assesses symptoms such as guilt, anxiety, and suicidal thoughts. Scores range from 0 to 30, with higher scores indicating a greater likelihood of PND.

While the EPDS is highly effective, it is not infallible. Some women may underreport symptoms due to shame or fear of consequences, such as being deemed unfit to care for their child. Other tools, like the Postpartum Depression Screening Scale (PDSS) or the Patient Health Questionnaire-9 (PHQ-9), may be used in conjunction to provide a more comprehensive assessment.

In clinical practice, these tools are often supplemented with a thorough clinical interview. A healthcare provider might explore the duration and severity of symptoms, their impact on daily functioning, and any history of depression or anxiety. Real-life application of these tools can be seen in cases like Sarah's, a first-time mother who scored moderately on the EPDS but revealed during her interview that she had been hiding intense feelings of worthlessness. This additional context allowed her provider to recommend targeted treatment rather than dismissing her struggles as fleeting "baby blues."

Challenges in Diagnosis

Despite the availability of screening tools, diagnosing postnatal depression is far from straightforward. One major hurdle is the overlap between PND symptoms and the typical exhaustion and emotional volatility of new motherhood. Sleep deprivation, for example, can mimic depression, making it difficult to discern where normal adjustment ends and clinical depression begins.

Cultural and societal factors further complicate the picture. In some communities, mental health struggles are stigmatized, leading women to suffer in silence rather than seek help. Others may fear that admitting to PND will result in their child being taken away, a misconception that prevents many from speaking openly with healthcare providers.

Language barriers and lack of access to culturally competent care can also delay diagnosis. For immigrant women or those from marginalized backgrounds, finding a provider who understands their unique cultural context is often a challenge. These systemic barriers underscore the need for more inclusive and accessible mental health services.

Overcoming Stigma and Seeking Help

The stigma surrounding postnatal depression is one of the most significant barriers to diagnosis and treatment. Many women internalize societal expectations that motherhood should be effortless and joyous, leaving them feeling isolated and ashamed when their reality falls short. Breaking this cycle requires both individual and collective action.

For mothers struggling with PND, the first step is acknowledging that seeking help is a sign of strength, not weakness. Support groups, whether in-person or online, can provide a sense of community and validation. Organizations like Postpartum Support International offer resources and connections to trained professionals who specialize in maternal mental health.

Family and friends also play a crucial role in reducing stigma. Simple acts of listening without judgment, offering practical help with childcare, or encouraging a loved one to attend a therapy session can make a profound difference. Education is key—dispelling myths about PND and framing it as a treatable medical condition rather than a personal failing can empower women to seek the care they need.

Case Studies and Real-Life Experiences

Real stories of women who have navigated postnatal depression can offer hope and practical insights. Take, for example, Maria, a mother of two who initially dismissed her fatigue and irritability as normal postpartum stress. It wasn't until her partner noticed her withdrawing from family life that she agreed to see a therapist. With a combination of counseling and medication, Maria gradually regained her sense of self and joy in motherhood.

Then there's Aisha, who faced cultural pressure to appear "strong" for her family. She hid her symptoms until a routine pediatric visit included a depression screening. Her pediatrician's compassionate approach helped her realize that her struggles were valid and treatable. These stories highlight the importance of persistence, support, and professional intervention in the journey to recovery.

Conclusion

Diagnosing postnatal depression is a multifaceted process that requires awareness, empathy, and proactive engagement from both healthcare providers and mothers themselves. While challenges like stigma and symptom overlap persist, the growing recognition of PND as a serious and treatable condition offers hope. By leveraging screening tools, fostering open communication, and dismantling societal barriers, we can ensure that no mother has to suffer in silence.

If you or someone you know is experiencing symptoms of PND, remember: reaching out for help is the first step toward healing. You are not alone, and with the right support, recovery is not just possible—it's within reach.

Treatment Options Overview

Chapter 4: Treatment Options Overview

Postnatal depression (PND) affects approximately one in seven women, yet it remains shrouded in silence and stigma. The journey to recovery can feel overwhelming, especially when faced with the demands of new motherhood. However, understanding the range of treatment options available is the first step toward reclaiming your mental well-being. This chapter provides a comprehensive overview of evidence-based treatments, from psychotherapy and medication to alternative therapies and combination approaches. By exploring these pathways, you'll gain the knowledge and confidence to make informed decisions about your care.

Psychotherapy: A Path to Healing

Psychotherapy is one of the most effective treatments for postnatal depression, offering a safe space to process emotions, develop coping strategies, and rebuild self-esteem. Two of the most widely researched and recommended therapies for PND are cognitive-behavioral therapy (CBT) and interpersonal therapy (IPT).

Cognitive-behavioral therapy focuses on identifying and challenging negative thought patterns that contribute to depression. For new mothers, these might include feelings of inadequacy, guilt, or fear of failure. A

CBT therapist will help you reframe these thoughts and adopt healthier perspectives. Practical exercises, such as journaling or behavioral activation, can be integrated into daily life to reinforce progress.

Interpersonal therapy, on the other hand, centers on improving relationships and addressing role transitions—key factors in PND. Becoming a mother often brings significant shifts in identity, social dynamics, and emotional support systems. IPT helps you navigate these changes, strengthen communication with partners and family, and reduce feelings of isolation.

Finding the right therapist is crucial. Look for professionals with experience in perinatal mental health, and don't hesitate to ask about their approach during an initial consultation. Many therapists offer virtual sessions, which can be a lifeline for busy mothers. Consistency is key; even if progress feels slow, regular sessions build a foundation for lasting recovery.

Medication: What You Need to Know

For some women, medication is an essential component of PND treatment. Antidepressants, particularly selective serotonin reuptake inhibitors (SSRIs), are commonly prescribed and have been shown to alleviate symptoms effectively. However, the decision to use medication is deeply personal and often comes with questions and concerns.

One of the most pressing concerns for new mothers is the safety of antidepressants while breastfeeding. The good news is that many SSRIs, such as sertraline, are considered compatible with breastfeeding, with minimal risk to the infant. Your healthcare provider can guide you in selecting a medication that balances efficacy and safety.

Side effects, such as nausea, dizziness, or fatigue, are possible but often subside within a few weeks. It's important to communicate openly with your doctor about any concerns, as dosage adjustments or alternative medications may be necessary. Hormonal treatments, such as estrogen therapy, are sometimes explored for PND linked to dramatic hormonal shifts, though research in this area is still evolving.

Medication is not a one-size-fits-all solution, and it works best when combined with other therapies. If you choose this route, give yourself permission to prioritize your mental health—your well-being is just as important as your baby's.

Alternative Therapies: Holistic Approaches

For those seeking non-pharmacological options or complementary treatments, alternative therapies offer a range of benefits. Mindfulness practices, such as meditation and deep-breathing exercises, can reduce stress and improve emotional regulation. Even five minutes of mindful breathing each day can make a difference.

Yoga, particularly postnatal yoga, combines physical movement with mental relaxation, helping to release tension and boost mood. Look for classes designed for new mothers, which often include baby-friendly modifications. Acupuncture, though less commonly discussed, has shown promise in reducing depressive symptoms by balancing the body's energy flow.

Dietary changes can also play a role. Nutrient deficiencies, particularly in omega-3 fatty acids, vitamin D, and B vitamins, have been linked to mood disorders. Incorporating foods like fatty fish, leafy greens, and nuts can support brain health. While diet alone isn't a cure, it's a valuable piece of the recovery puzzle.

The key to success with alternative therapies is consistency and patience. Start small—perhaps with a short daily meditation or a weekly yoga class—and gradually build a routine that feels sustainable.

Combination Treatments: Maximizing Recovery

The most effective treatment plans often integrate multiple approaches. Combining psychotherapy, medication, and alternative therapies can address PND from different angles, enhancing overall recovery. For example, a woman might use CBT to manage negative thoughts, an SSRI to stabilize mood, and yoga to reduce physical tension.

Case studies highlight the power of combination treatments. Sarah, a mother of two, struggled with severe PND after her second child. Therapy helped her process unresolved grief, while medication provided the stability she needed to engage fully in sessions. Adding mindfulness exercises gave her tools to cope with daily stressors. Over time, this multifaceted approach led to significant improvement.

Creating a personalized plan requires collaboration with healthcare providers. Be open about your preferences and concerns, and don't be afraid to adjust your strategy as needed. Recovery is not linear, and flexibility is essential.

Overcoming Stigma and Seeking Support

Despite its prevalence, postnatal depression is often misunderstood or dismissed. Many women fear judgment or worry they'll be labeled as "bad mothers." Breaking through this stigma starts with honest conversations. Share your experience with trusted friends or family members—you might be surprised by their support.

Support groups, whether in-person or online, connect you with others who understand your struggles. Organizations like Postpartum Support International offer resources and directories of local groups. Advocacy is also powerful; by speaking openly about PND, you help normalize the conversation and pave the way for better mental health care.

Remember, seeking help is a sign of strength, not weakness. You deserve support, and reaching out is the first step toward healing.

Conclusion

Postnatal depression is treatable, and you are not alone in this journey. From psychotherapy and medication to holistic practices and combination treatments, there are multiple pathways to recovery. The best approach is one that aligns with your unique needs, preferences, and circumstances.

Take the insights from this chapter and use them to advocate for your mental health. Whether you start with therapy, explore medication, or incorporate mindfulness into your routine, each step forward is a victory. With the right support and resources, you can overcome PND and embrace the joy of motherhood with renewed strength and resilience.

The road to recovery begins with a single step—take it today.

5

Medication and PND

Chapter 5: Medication and PND

Postnatal Depression (PND) is a complex and deeply personal experience that affects many women during what is often portrayed as one of the happiest times of their lives. For those grappling with PND, medication can be a vital component of a holistic treatment plan, offering relief from symptoms and paving the way for recovery. However, deciding to take medication—particularly as a new mother—can feel overwhelming. This chapter aims to demystify the role of medication in treating PND, providing you with the knowledge and tools to make informed decisions about your mental health while balancing the needs of your baby.

Understanding Medication as a Treatment Option

Medication is one of several treatment options available for PND, often used in conjunction with therapy, lifestyle changes, and support networks. It is not a one-size-fits-all solution, but for many women, it can be a game-changer in managing symptoms such as persistent sadness, anxiety, fatigue, and difficulty bonding with their baby. Medication works by restoring chemical imbalances in the brain, helping to stabilize mood and improve overall well-being.

Despite its potential benefits, medication is sometimes stigmatized, with misconceptions suggesting that it is a sign of weakness or a last resort. It's important to recognize that seeking help and considering medication is a courageous and proactive step toward recovery. Research shows that medication, when prescribed appropriately, can significantly reduce symptoms of PND and improve quality of life. Consulting a healthcare professional is essential to determine whether medication is right for you, as they can tailor treatment to your specific needs and circumstances.

Types of Medications for PND

Several types of medications are commonly prescribed for PND, each targeting different symptoms and underlying causes. Understanding these options can help you feel more confident in discussing treatment with your healthcare provider.

Antidepressants are the most widely used medications for PND. Selective Serotonin Reuptake Inhibitors (SSRIs), such as sertraline and fluoxetine, are often the first line of treatment. SSRIs work by increasing levels of serotonin, a neurotransmitter that regulates mood, in the brain. They are generally effective, well-tolerated, and have fewer side effects compared to older antidepressants. Another option is Serotonin and Norepinephrine Reuptake Inhibitors (SNRIs), which target both serotonin and norepinephrine, another mood-regulating chemical.

Anti-anxiety medications, such as benzodiazepines, may be prescribed for women experiencing severe anxiety alongside depression. These medications provide short-term relief but are typically not recommended for long-term use due to the risk of dependency. Hormone-based treatments, such as estrogen therapy, are less commonly prescribed but may be considered for women whose PND is linked to hormonal fluctuations.

The dosage and duration of treatment vary depending on the individual. Some women may start to feel better within a few weeks, while others may require several months of treatment. It's important to follow your healthcare provider's guidance and avoid stopping medication abruptly, as this can lead to withdrawal symptoms or a relapse of depression.

Benefits and Risks of Medication

Like all medical treatments, medication for PND comes with both benefits and risks. Understanding these can help you make an informed decision and manage your treatment effectively.

The primary benefit of medication is its ability to alleviate symptoms of PND, allowing you to function more effectively and engage more fully in your daily life. For many women, medication provides the stability needed to participate in therapy, build a support network, and develop coping strategies. It can also improve sleep, energy levels, and overall mood, making it easier to care for your baby and yourself.

However, medication is not without potential risks. Common side effects of antidepressants include nausea, dizziness, headaches, and changes in appetite or sleep patterns. These side effects are usually mild and tend to diminish over time as your body adjusts to the medication. More serious side effects, such as increased suicidal thoughts, are rare but should be discussed with your healthcare provider if they occur.

Long-term use of medication may require regular monitoring to ensure its continued effectiveness and safety. Some women may experience withdrawal symptoms if they discontinue medication too quickly, so it's important to work with your healthcare provider to taper off gradually if needed. Open communication with your provider is key to managing side effects and making adjustments to your treatment plan as necessary.

Medication and Breastfeeding: What You Need to Know

For breastfeeding mothers, the decision to take medication can be particularly challenging. The good news is that many medications are compatible with breastfeeding, allowing you to prioritize both your mental health and your baby's well-being.

Research shows that SSRIs like sertraline are generally safe during lactation, with minimal transfer to breast milk and low risk to the infant. Your healthcare provider can help you choose a medication that balances effectiveness with safety for your baby. It's important to discuss any concerns you have and to monitor your baby for potential side effects, such as drowsiness or irritability, although these are rare.

If you prefer to avoid medication or are concerned about its impact on breastfeeding, alternative treatments such as therapy, lifestyle changes, and support groups can be effective. However, for some women, medication is necessary to manage severe symptoms of PND. In such cases, continuing to breastfeed while taking medication is often possible and can be supported by guidance from your healthcare provider.

Practical tips for balancing breastfeeding and medication include timing doses to minimize exposure, staying informed about the latest research, and seeking support from lactation consultants or mental health professionals. Remember, your mental health is just as important as your baby's physical health, and finding a treatment plan that works for both is achievable.

Making an Informed Decision

Deciding whether to take medication for PND is a deeply personal choice that requires careful consideration of your unique circumstances. By weighing the benefits and risks, consulting healthcare professionals, and considering your preferences and values, you can make an informed decision that prioritizes your well-being and that of your baby.

It's important to advocate for yourself and communicate openly with your healthcare provider about your concerns, goals, and preferences. Treatment for PND is not a one-size-fits-all approach, and finding the right combination of therapies may take time. Be patient with yourself and trust that seeking help is a positive step toward recovery.

Remember, you are not alone in this journey. Many women have navigated PND and found effective treatments that allowed them to regain their sense of self and enjoy motherhood. By taking an active role in your mental health care, you are setting a powerful example of strength and resilience for yourself and your family.

Conclusion

Medication can be a valuable tool in treating Postnatal Depression, offering relief from symptoms and helping you regain balance during a challenging time. By understanding the types of medications available, their benefits and risks, and the considerations for breastfeeding mothers, you can make informed decisions about your treatment. Remember, seeking help is a sign of strength, and prioritizing your mental health is essential for both you and your baby. With the right support and treatment, recovery from PND is possible, allowing you to embrace motherhood with confidence and joy.

6

Psychotherapy Approaches

Chapter 6: Psychotherapy Approaches

Postnatal depression (PND) is a complex and deeply personal experience, but it is important to remember that it is also treatable. Among the most effective treatments available are psychotherapy approaches, which provide structured, evidence-based methods for addressing the emotional, cognitive, and relational challenges that often accompany PND. This chapter explores the most widely recommended therapies—Cognitive Behavioral Therapy (CBT) and Interpersonal Therapy (IPT)—along with the invaluable role of support groups. It also addresses societal stigma and offers guidance on creating a personalized treatment plan. By understanding these options, you can take informed steps toward healing and reclaiming your sense of self during this transformative period.

Understanding Cognitive Behavioral Therapy (CBT)

Cognitive Behavioral Therapy (CBT) is one of the most widely researched and proven therapies for treating postnatal depression. It operates on the principle that our thoughts, feelings, and behaviors are interconnected. For women experiencing PND, negative thought patterns—such as feelings of inadequacy, guilt, or hopelessness—can exacerbate emotional distress. CBT works by helping individuals identify these unhelpful thoughts, challenge their validity, and replace them with more balanced and constructive alternatives.

A key component of CBT is cognitive restructuring, a technique that involves examining the evidence for and against negative beliefs. For example, a new mother might think, "I'm a terrible parent because I can't soothe my baby." A therapist trained in CBT would guide her to explore this belief, asking questions like, "What evidence supports this thought? Is there evidence that contradicts it?" Through this process, she might recognize that while parenting is challenging, she is doing her best and learning as she goes.

Another important aspect of CBT is behavioral activation, which encourages individuals to engage in activities that bring a sense of accomplishment or joy. For mothers with PND, this might involve setting small, achievable goals, such as taking a short walk outside or spending 10 minutes on a hobby. These activities can help break the cycle of inactivity and low mood that often accompanies depression.

Research consistently shows that CBT is effective in reducing PND symptoms, with many women experiencing significant improvement within 12 to 16 sessions. To find a qualified CBT therapist, consider asking your healthcare provider for a referral or searching for licensed professionals through reputable organizations such as the Association for Behavioral and Cognitive Therapies (ABCT).

The Role of Interpersonal Therapy (IPT)

Interpersonal Therapy (IPT) is another evidence-based approach that focuses on improving relationships and communication skills. For many women, the transition to motherhood can strain relationships with partners, family members, or friends, leading to feelings of loneliness and conflict. IPT addresses these challenges by helping individuals navigate four key problem areas: grief, role transitions, interpersonal disputes, and social isolation.

Grief is a common focus in IPT, particularly for women who may be mourning the loss of their pre-parenthood identity or grappling with unmet expectations about motherhood. Role transitions, such as adjusting to the demands of caring for a newborn, can also be a source of stress. IPT helps individuals process these changes and develop strategies for adapting to their new roles.

Interpersonal disputes, whether with a partner or family member, are another area of focus. IPT emphasizes effective communication techniques, such as active listening and expressing needs clearly, to resolve conflicts and strengthen relationships. Finally, social isolation—a common experience for new mothers—is addressed by encouraging individuals to rebuild connections and seek support from their social networks.

Case studies highlight the effectiveness of IPT in reducing PND symptoms. For example, one mother struggling with feelings of resentment toward her partner found that IPT helped her articulate her needs and work collaboratively to distribute parenting responsibilities. Another woman, who felt disconnected from her friends after becoming a mother, used IPT to rebuild these relationships by scheduling regular catch-ups and being open about her experiences.

To explore IPT, look for therapists trained in this modality through professional organizations like the International Society for Interpersonal Psychotherapy (ISIPT).

The Power of Support Groups

While individual therapy offers personalized support, support groups provide a communal space where women can share their experiences, receive emotional validation, and gain practical advice. For many mothers, realizing that they are not alone in their struggles can be profoundly comforting. Support groups reduce feelings of isolation and foster a sense of belonging, which is especially important during the often overwhelming postpartum period.

Support groups can take various forms, including in-person meetings, online forums, and social media communities. Some groups are facilitated by mental health professionals, while others are peer-led. When choosing a group, consider factors such as the group's focus (e.g., general PND, specific challenges like breastfeeding or sleep deprivation) and the facilitator's qualifications.

Common concerns about attending support groups include worries about privacy and judgment. It's important to remember that reputable groups prioritize confidentiality and create a non-judgmental atmosphere. Many women find that once they overcome their initial hesitation, the benefits of participation far outweigh their fears.

To find a support group, ask your healthcare provider for recommendations or search online resources like Postpartum Support International (PSI). Local community centers and hospitals may also host groups.

Overcoming Societal Stigma

Unfortunately, societal stigma surrounding postnatal depression persists, often preventing women from seeking the help they need. Misconceptions—such as the belief that PND is a sign of weakness or that mothers should be able to "snap out of it"—can exacerbate feelings of shame and isolation. However, seeking help is a sign of strength and self-awareness, not weakness.

To combat stigma, educate yourself and others about PND. Share reliable information with family members and friends to foster understanding and support. Advocate for better mental health resources in your community by participating in awareness campaigns or supporting organizations that promote maternal mental health.

Research shows that reducing stigma improves treatment outcomes by encouraging more women to seek help early. By openly discussing your experiences and challenging stereotypes, you can contribute to a more supportive environment for all mothers.

Creating a Personalized Treatment Plan

Every woman's experience with PND is unique, which is why a personalized treatment plan is essential. Collaboration between you and your healthcare provider is key to developing a plan that addresses your specific needs and preferences. This plan may incorporate a combination of therapies, medication, and lifestyle changes.

To create an effective plan, start by identifying your primary challenges and goals. Are you struggling with overwhelming sadness? Difficulty bonding with your baby? Conflict in your relationships? Clearly defining your priorities will help guide your treatment decisions.

Track your progress regularly, noting any changes in mood, behavior, or relationships. This information can help you and your therapist adjust your plan as needed. Set achievable goals, such as attending therapy sessions consistently or practicing self-care daily, and celebrate small victories along the way.

Maintaining open communication with your therapist or healthcare provider is crucial. Don't hesitate to share any concerns or ask questions about your treatment. Remember, recovery is a journey, and it's okay to seek support along the way.

Conclusion

Postnatal depression is a challenging but treatable condition, and psychotherapy offers powerful tools for healing and growth. Whether you choose Cognitive Behavioral Therapy, Interpersonal Therapy, or a support group, each approach provides unique benefits that can help you navigate the complexities of PND. Overcoming societal stigma and creating a personalized treatment plan are equally important steps in your journey toward recovery.

Remember, seeking help is a courageous act, and you don't have to face this alone. By taking informed, proactive steps, you can regain your sense of balance and joy during this transformative period. Your well-being matters, and with the right support, you can emerge stronger and more resilient than ever.

7

Impact on Family Dynamics

Chapter 7: Impact on Family Dynamics

Postnatal depression (PND) is often perceived as an individual struggle, but its effects ripple outward, reshaping relationships and altering the emotional landscape of the entire family. Partners, children, and extended family members all find themselves navigating uncharted territory, grappling with feelings of confusion, frustration, and helplessness. This chapter explores the profound ways PND impacts family dynamics, offering practical strategies to foster understanding, resilience, and healing. By acknowledging these challenges and providing actionable solutions, families can emerge stronger, more connected, and better equipped to support one another.

The Strain on Partners: Navigating Emotional Turbulence

When a mother experiences PND, her partner often becomes the primary source of support—a role that can be both emotionally and physically exhausting. Many partners report feelings of helplessness, frustration, and even loneliness as they struggle to understand what their loved one is going through. Research shows that PND can strain communication, reduce intimacy, and create a sense of emotional distance in relationships.

One of the most common challenges partners face is the inability to "fix" the situation. Unlike physical ailments, PND doesn't have a straightforward solution, which can leave partners feeling powerless. This frustration can sometimes manifest as impatience or withdrawal, further isolating the mother when she needs connection the most.

To navigate these challenges, partners must prioritize empathy and teamwork. Open communication is essential; setting aside time to talk honestly about emotions—without judgment—can help bridge the gap. Practical support, such as sharing household responsibilities or arranging childcare to give the mother a break, can also alleviate stress. Additionally, partners should not neglect their own mental health. Seeking individual therapy or joining a support group can provide much-needed emotional relief and perspective.

Case studies of couples who successfully weathered PND highlight the importance of patience and mutual effort. One couple, for example, implemented a nightly "check-in" ritual where they shared their highs and lows of the day. This simple practice helped them stay emotionally connected even during the darkest moments.

Children in the Shadow: Understanding the Impact on Kids

Children, even very young ones, are acutely sensitive to their mother's emotional state. While infants may not understand PND, they can pick up on changes in their mother's mood, responsiveness, and energy levels. Research suggests that prolonged exposure to a mother's untreated PND can influence a child's emotional development, attachment style, and even behavior.

For infants, inconsistent caregiving due to PND may lead to attachment issues, manifesting as clinginess or difficulty self-soothing. Toddlers and preschoolers might exhibit regressive behaviors, such as bedwetting or tantrums, as they struggle to process the shift in their mother's demeanor. Older children may internalize their confusion, blaming themselves for their mother's sadness or withdrawing emotionally.

Mitigating these effects requires intentional effort. Maintaining routines—bedtimes, meals, and playtime—can provide children with a sense of stability. Simple, age-appropriate explanations, such as "Mommy is feeling sad right now, but it's not your fault," can help alleviate guilt or confusion. Partners and other caregivers should step in to ensure children continue receiving affection and attention, even when the mother is struggling.

One mother shared how her partner took over bedtime stories when she was too exhausted, ensuring their child still felt loved and secure. Over time, as she recovered, she reintegrated into these routines, rebuilding their bond gradually.

Rebuilding Family Bonds: Practical Support Strategies

Recovery from PND is a collective effort, requiring the entire family to work together. Establishing a strong support network is crucial—whether it's leaning on extended family, friends, or professional services. Practical steps, such as meal trains or shared childcare duties, can ease daily pressures, allowing the mother to focus on healing.

Open communication within the family is equally important. Regular family meetings, where everyone can express their feelings in a safe space, foster understanding and unity. Encouraging children to share their emotions through art or play can also help them process complex feelings.

Professional help should not be overlooked. Family therapy can provide a structured environment to address unresolved tensions and develop healthy coping mechanisms. Individual therapy for the mother, and sometimes the partner, can also be invaluable in navigating the emotional fallout of PND.

A case study of one family's recovery highlights the power of small, consistent actions. They created a "gratitude jar," where each family member dropped notes about things they appreciated about one another. Over time, this practice helped shift their focus from frustration to connection.

Breaking the Stigma: Addressing Societal Misconceptions

Societal stigma surrounding PND often compounds the challenges families face. Misconceptions—such as the belief that PND is simply "baby blues" or a sign of weakness—can make mothers reluctant to seek help. Partners may also downplay the severity of the condition, believing it will resolve on its own.

Combatting this stigma starts with education. Families can benefit from learning about PND's biological and psychological roots, which helps normalize the experience. Sharing personal stories, whether privately with friends or publicly through advocacy, can also chip away at societal shame.

Mental health advocates emphasize the importance of language. Phrases like "Just snap out of it" or "You should be happy" are not only unhelpful but harmful. Instead, offering validation—"This must be so hard, but you're not alone"—can make a world of difference.

Looking Ahead: Long-Term Family Recovery and Growth

While PND is undeniably challenging, many families find that navigating it together strengthens their bonds in unexpected ways. The key to long-term recovery lies in patience, forgiveness, and ongoing communication. Families should celebrate small victories, whether it's a good day for the mother or a moment of connection between parent and child.

Continuing to prioritize mental health beyond the immediate crisis is essential. Regular check-ins, maintaining therapy if needed, and fostering a culture of openness can prevent future relapses and ensure lasting emotional well-being.

One family's story stands out: after years of struggling with PND, they emerged with a deeper appreciation for one another. They now volunteer together at a maternal mental health organization, turning their pain into purpose.

Conclusion

Postnatal depression reshapes family dynamics, but it doesn't have to define them. By understanding its impact on partners and children, implementing practical support strategies, and challenging societal stigma, families can navigate this difficult journey with resilience. The road to recovery may be long, but with empathy, teamwork, and professional guidance, families can not only heal but grow stronger together. The stories of those who have walked this path serve as a powerful reminder: even in the darkest moments, hope and connection are possible.

8

Societal Stigma and Mental Health

Chapter 8: Societal Stigma and Mental Health

The journey into motherhood is often painted in hues of joy, fulfillment, and unconditional love. Yet for many women, the reality is far more complex, marked by emotional turbulence, exhaustion, and, in some cases, the debilitating weight of postnatal depression (PND). While PND affects approximately one in seven new mothers, societal stigma continues to silence conversations around it, leaving women to suffer in isolation. This chapter explores the pervasive stigma surrounding postnatal depression, examining how cultural perceptions, media portrayals, and societal biases create barriers to seeking help. More importantly, it offers actionable strategies for breaking down these barriers, fostering a more compassionate and inclusive environment for mothers navigating PND.

Cultural Perceptions of Postnatal Depression

Cultural beliefs and traditions play a significant role in shaping attitudes toward postnatal depression. In some societies, motherhood is idealized as a natural and effortless transition, leaving little room for discussions about mental health struggles. Women who admit to feeling overwhelmed or depressed after childbirth may face judgment, dismissal, or even accusations of being unfit mothers.

For example, in many Western cultures, there is an expectation that new mothers should embody resilience and self-sacrifice, often discouraging them from voicing their struggles. Conversely, in some Asian and African communities, postnatal emotional distress may be attributed to spiritual or supernatural causes rather than recognized as a medical condition. These cultural narratives can prevent women from seeking professional help, as they fear being labeled as weak or ungrateful.

However, cultural contexts are not monolithic. Some societies have built-in support systems that naturally mitigate the effects of PND. In countries like Japan, the tradition of *satogaeri bunben*—where mothers return to their family homes for postpartum care—provides built-in emotional and practical support. Similarly, Latin American cultures often emphasize communal care during the *cuarentena*, a 40-day period of rest and recovery. These examples highlight how cultural practices can either exacerbate or alleviate the stigma surrounding PND.

For women navigating cultural barriers, education and open dialogue are key. Encouraging conversations about mental health within families and communities can help shift perceptions. Partnering with cultural leaders, healthcare providers, and advocacy groups to normalize discussions around PND is another powerful step. By reframing postnatal depression as a common and treatable condition—rather than a personal failing—we can begin to dismantle the cultural stigma that silences so many women.

Media Portrayal and Its Influence on Stigma

The media wields immense power in shaping public perception, and its portrayal of postnatal depression has often been fraught with inaccuracies and sensationalism. Popular films and television shows frequently depict mothers with PND as unstable, dangerous, or even villainous, reinforcing harmful stereotypes. Headlines that focus on extreme cases—such as postpartum psychosis—without proper context further distort the public's understanding of PND as a spectrum of experiences.

Yet, the media also holds the potential to be a force for good. Campaigns like *#SpeakThesecret* in the UK and *This Is My Brave* in the US have used storytelling to humanize postnatal depression, showcasing real women's experiences in an empathetic light. Documentaries such as *When the Bough Breaks* have brought scientific and personal perspectives to mainstream audiences, fostering greater awareness and understanding.

As consumers of media, we can advocate for more responsible portrayals of PND by supporting content that accurately represents the condition. Sharing personal stories on social media, writing to journalists about balanced reporting, and engaging with mental health organizations that promote accurate messaging are all ways to push back against harmful narratives. By demanding nuance and compassion in media portrayals, we can help shift the conversation from shame to support.

The Real-World Impact of Stigma on New Mothers

The consequences of societal stigma are not abstract—they have real and profound effects on women's lives. Many mothers with PND report feeling intense shame, believing they are failing at the one role society tells them should come naturally. This shame often leads to isolation, as women withdraw from friends and family to avoid judgment. Worse still, the fear of being seen as an inadequate mother can deter women from seeking professional help, delaying critical treatment.

Research underscores the toll of this stigma. Studies show that women who internalize negative societal attitudes about PND experience higher levels of guilt and lower self-esteem, exacerbating their symptoms. In extreme cases, untreated postnatal depression can lead to severe emotional distress, strained relationships, and even self-harm.

Personal stories bring these statistics to life. Take Maria, a first-time mother who hid her struggles for months, fearing her family would see her as "broken." Or Aisha, who was told by her community that her depression was a sign of spiritual weakness, leaving her feeling utterly alone. These narratives highlight the urgent need for societal change—one where no mother feels compelled to suffer in silence.

Practical strategies can help mitigate the impact of stigma. Peer support groups, whether in-person or online, provide safe spaces for women to share their experiences without fear of judgment. Mental health advocacy organizations often offer resources and helplines for those in need. Simply knowing that they are not alone can be a lifeline for mothers grappling with PND.

Breaking Down Stigma: Steps Toward Change

Dismantling the stigma surrounding postnatal depression requires collective effort. Education is the foundation of this change—dispelling myths, providing accurate information, and normalizing conversations about mental health. Workshops in schools, workplaces, and community centers can equip people with the knowledge to support new mothers compassionately.

Open dialogue is equally crucial. Encouraging mothers to speak openly about their experiences—and listening without judgment—helps break the cycle of silence. Social media campaigns, blogs, and public speaking opportunities amplify these voices, demonstrating that PND is neither rare nor shameful.

Policy changes also play a vital role. Advocacy for better maternal mental health care, including mandatory screening for PND and improved access to therapy, can save lives. Employers can support new mothers by offering flexible work arrangements and mental health days. Governments and healthcare systems must prioritize funding for PND research and treatment programs.

On an individual level, everyone has a role to play. If you know a new mother, check in on her—not just with a casual "How are you?" but with genuine curiosity and empathy. Challenge stigmatizing language when you hear it. Share resources and stories that promote understanding. Small actions, multiplied across communities, can create a seismic shift in how society views postnatal depression.

Conclusion

The stigma surrounding postnatal depression is a formidable barrier, but it is not insurmountable. By examining cultural perceptions, holding the media accountable, and understanding the real-world impact of stigma, we can begin to foster a more supportive environment for new mothers. Change starts with education, empathy, and the courage to speak openly about mental health.

No mother should have to navigate postnatal depression alone. Together, we can replace silence with support, shame with understanding, and stigma with solidarity. The journey toward mental wellness is not just an individual one—it is a collective responsibility, and it begins with each of us.

9

Building a Support Network

Chapter 9: Building a Support Network

The journey through postnatal depression (PND) can feel isolating and overwhelming, but no mother should have to face it alone. Building a strong support network is one of the most effective ways to navigate the challenges of PND and foster recovery. A support network provides emotional reassurance, practical assistance, and a sense of belonging, all of which are essential for healing. This chapter explores the critical role of friends and family, the value of community resources, and the growing influence of online support communities. It also offers practical advice on how to build, maintain, and advocate for a support system tailored to your unique needs.

The Role of Friends and Family

Friends and family often serve as the first line of support for women experiencing postnatal depression. Their role in providing emotional comfort and practical help cannot be overstated. Loved ones can offer a listening ear, validate your feelings, and remind you that you are not alone. They can also assist with daily tasks such as childcare, cooking, or cleaning, easing the burden during a challenging time.

However, navigating PND with friends and family can also present challenges. Misunderstandings about PND are common, and well-meaning loved ones may struggle to know how best to help. Open and honest communication is key. Share your feelings and needs clearly, and don't hesitate to educate those around you about PND. Phrases like "I'm feeling overwhelmed right now" or "I could really use your help with..." can guide your loved ones in providing meaningful support.

Case studies highlight the transformative power of family support. Take Sarah, for example, a new mother who struggled with PND after the birth of her second child. Initially, her husband didn't understand the severity of her symptoms and assumed she would simply "snap out of it." After Sarah attended a parenting workshop on PND, she shared what she learned with her husband. This opened the door to honest conversations, and together they developed a plan to share responsibilities and prioritize her mental health. Over time, their teamwork not only helped Sarah recover but also strengthened their relationship.

Friends, too, can play a vital role. Emily, a single mother, leaned on her close friend Jessica during her PND journey. Jessica regularly checked in on Emily, brought her meals, and even helped her find a therapist. Their friendship became a lifeline, demonstrating how small acts of kindness can make a profound difference.

Community Resources for New Mothers

Beyond friends and family, community resources offer invaluable support for mothers experiencing PND. Maternal wellness programs, support groups, and healthcare services tailored to postnatal mental health can provide professional guidance and a sense of community. These resources are designed to address the unique challenges of motherhood and PND, offering practical tools and emotional reassurance.

To access these resources, start by researching local organizations and healthcare providers. Many hospitals and clinics offer postnatal mental health services, including counseling and therapy groups. Community centers and nonprofits often host maternal wellness programs, such as yoga classes, parenting workshops, and peer support groups. Online directories and social media platforms can help you identify options in your area.

When evaluating these resources, consider factors such as accessibility, affordability, and alignment with your needs. Don't hesitate to reach out to program coordinators or facilitators with questions. Many mothers find it helpful to attend a trial session or meet with a counselor before committing to a program.

Successful community initiatives illustrate the impact of these resources. For instance, the "Motherhood Matters" program in Chicago offers free weekly support groups led by licensed therapists. Participants report feeling less isolated and more empowered to manage their PND symptoms. Similarly, the "Postnatal Wellness Hub" in London provides holistic care, combining therapy, nutrition guidance, and childcare support. These programs demonstrate how tailored community resources can transform mothers' mental health and well-being.

The Power of Online Support Communities

In today's digital age, online support communities have emerged as a vital resource for women with PND. These virtual spaces offer accessibility, anonymity, and inclusivity, making them an attractive option for mothers who may feel overwhelmed or stigmatized in traditional settings. Online forums, social media groups, and apps like Peanut and MomCo connect mothers with peers who share similar experiences, fostering a sense of solidarity and understanding.

The benefits of online support are immense. Many mothers appreciate the ability to access support at any time of day or night, particularly during sleepless nights or moments of crisis. Virtual connections also allow women to share their stories openly without fear of judgment, creating a safe space for vulnerability and healing.

However, online communities also come with potential drawbacks, such as misinformation or negative interactions. To navigate these challenges, seek out reputable groups moderated by professionals or experienced mothers. Verify the credibility of information shared online, and don't hesitate to consult healthcare providers for clarification. Setting boundaries around your online engagement can also help maintain a positive experience.

Case studies of popular online communities highlight their effectiveness. The "PND Warriors" Facebook group, for example, has grown into a global network of mothers supporting one another through PND. Members share coping strategies, celebrate milestones, and offer encouragement in times of struggle. The group's success lies in its emphasis on empathy and mutual respect, creating a nurturing environment for recovery.

Building and Maintaining Your Support Network

Creating a personalized support network requires intentionality and self-advocacy. Start by identifying the right mix of friends, family, community resources, and online groups to meet your needs. Consider factors such as proximity, availability, and compatibility with your values and personality. A diverse support system ensures that you have access to different types of assistance, whether it's emotional comfort, practical help, or professional guidance.

Once your network is in place, focus on maintaining it. Regular communication is essential—keep your loved ones informed about how you're feeling and what you need. Don't be afraid to ask for help, and remember that it's okay to lean on others during this time. Setting boundaries is equally important; prioritize your well-being by saying no to commitments that feel overwhelming.

Self-advocacy plays a crucial role in sustaining your support system. Educate yourself about PND and advocate for your mental health with healthcare providers and loved ones. Seek out resources that resonate with you, and don't hesitate to explore new options if your needs evolve. A strong support network is a dynamic, evolving entity that grows with you on your journey to recovery.

Conclusion

Building a support network is a powerful step toward overcoming postnatal depression. Friends and family, community resources, and online communities each play a unique role in providing the emotional and practical support needed for healing. By identifying and nurturing these connections, you can create a personalized network that empowers you to navigate PND with resilience and hope. Remember, you are not alone, and help is always within reach. Reach out, lean in, and embrace the strength of your support system as you move forward on your path to recovery.

10

Self-Care Strategies for New Mothers

Chapter 10: Self-Care Strategies for New Mothers

The journey into motherhood is one of the most transformative experiences a woman can undergo. However, it is also one of the most demanding, often leaving new mothers feeling exhausted, overwhelmed, and, in some cases, struggling with postnatal depression (PND). In the midst of caring for a newborn, many mothers neglect their own needs, believing that self-care is a luxury they cannot afford. This chapter emphasizes that self-care is not a luxury but a necessity, particularly for mothers dealing with PND. It offers practical strategies to integrate self-care into daily life, ensuring that mothers can prioritize their mental and physical health while fulfilling their parental responsibilities.

Understanding the Importance of Self-Care in PND

Self-care is often misunderstood as indulgent or selfish, when in reality, it is a vital component of mental health and well-being. For mothers experiencing postnatal depression, self-care becomes even more critical. PND is a complex condition that can manifest as persistent sadness, fatigue, irritability, and difficulty bonding with the baby. Without proper care, these symptoms can escalate, affecting both the mother and the child.

Research consistently shows that self-care plays a significant role in managing and reducing the symptoms of PND. Engaging in self-care practices can help regulate emotions, reduce stress, and improve overall mental health. Studies have found that mothers who prioritize self-care are less likely to experience severe depressive symptoms and are better equipped to handle the challenges of motherhood.

Self-care is not just about improving mental health; it also has a positive impact on physical health. Adequate sleep, proper nutrition, and regular exercise are essential components of self-care that can significantly reduce the risk of PND. When mothers take the time to care for themselves, they are better able to care for their babies, creating a positive cycle of well-being for both.

Practical Self-Care Strategies for New Mothers

Incorporating self-care into a busy motherhood routine may seem daunting, but it is entirely possible with a bit of planning and prioritization. Here are some practical strategies that mothers can implement to ensure they are caring for themselves while caring for their newborns.

First and foremost, sleep is crucial. Sleep deprivation can exacerbate the symptoms of PND, making it essential for mothers to find ways to rest whenever possible. While it may be challenging to get a full night's sleep with a newborn, mothers can take short naps during the day when the baby is sleeping. Creating a comfortable sleep environment and establishing a bedtime routine can also help improve sleep quality.

Setting aside 'me-time' is another vital aspect of self-care. This doesn't have to be a long period; even 10-15 minutes a day can make a difference. Mothers can use this time to engage in activities they enjoy, such as reading, meditating, or taking a relaxing bath. The key is to focus on activities that bring joy and relaxation, helping to recharge both the mind and body.

Physical activity is another powerful self-care tool. Exercise releases endorphins, which can alleviate symptoms of depression and boost mood. Mothers don't need to engage in intense workouts to reap the benefits; even a short walk or gentle yoga session can be effective. Incorporating physical activity into daily routines, such as taking the baby for a walk in the stroller, can also provide an opportunity for fresh air and social interaction.

Maintaining a healthy diet is equally important. Proper nutrition can have a significant impact on mental health, and mothers should aim to eat balanced meals with plenty of fruits, vegetables, lean proteins, and whole grains. Preparing meals in advance or accepting help with cooking can make it easier to maintain a healthy diet, especially on busy days.

Lastly, connecting with supportive communities can provide emotional support and reduce feelings of isolation. Mothers can join local or online parenting groups, participate in baby classes, or simply reach out to friends and family. Building a support network can offer reassurance and practical assistance, making motherhood a more manageable journey.

Balancing Motherhood and Self-Care

One of the biggest challenges mothers face is balancing their new responsibilities with the need for self-care. Many mothers feel guilty for prioritizing their own needs, fearing that it might detract from their ability to care for their baby. However, self-care is not selfish; it is essential for being the best parent possible.

The key to balancing motherhood and self-care lies in setting realistic expectations. Mothers should acknowledge that they cannot do everything perfectly and that it's okay to ask for help. Delegating tasks, whether to a partner, family member, or friend, can free up time for self-care activities. It's important to remember that taking care of oneself is ultimately beneficial for the baby, as a healthy and happy mother is better able to provide care and support.

Prioritizing self-care also involves learning to say no. Mothers often feel pressured to fulfill every social obligation or household chore, but it's important to recognize when these commitments are becoming too overwhelming. Saying no to unnecessary demands can create space for more meaningful self-care practices.

Incorporating self-care into daily routines can also help make it a consistent habit. For example, mothers can combine activities, such as listening to an audiobook while nursing or practicing mindfulness exercises while the baby naps. Finding small moments throughout the day to focus on self-care can make a significant difference over time.

Case Studies: Real-Life Applications

Hearing from other mothers who have successfully managed PND through self-care can provide valuable insights and inspiration. Here are two case studies that illustrate the practical application of self-care strategies and their positive outcomes.

Emma, a 32-year-old first-time mother, struggled with severe PND after the birth of her daughter. She felt overwhelmed, exhausted, and disconnected from her baby. With the support of her partner and therapist, Emma began incorporating self-care into her daily routine. She started by setting a goal to take short naps whenever possible, which helped reduce her fatigue. She also began attending a local parenting group, where she met other mothers who provided emotional support and practical advice. Over time, Emma's symptoms improved, and she felt more confident in her ability to care for her baby.

Sarah, a 28-year-old mother of twin boys, found herself juggling multiple responsibilities while battling PND. She felt guilty for taking time for herself, but her therapist emphasized the importance of self-care for her mental health. Sarah began scheduling 'me-time' into her day, even if it was just 10 minutes of meditation or a quick walk around the block. She also prioritized her diet, preparing healthy meals in advance to ensure she was eating well. With these changes, Sarah noticed a significant improvement in her mood and energy levels, allowing her to be more present and engaged with her sons.

Moving Forward: Maintaining Self-Care Practices

Maintaining self-care practices over the long term requires adaptability and commitment. As the child grows and the mother's lifestyle changes, it's important to reassess and adjust the self-care routine to ensure it remains effective and feasible.

For example, as the baby starts sleeping through the night, mothers can focus on getting more consistent sleep. As the child becomes more independent, mothers can explore new self-care activities, such as returning to hobbies or joining exercise classes. Regularly evaluating what works and what doesn't can help mothers stay on track with their self-care goals.

It's also essential to recognize that self-care is an ongoing process, not a one-time event. There will be periods when self-care feels more challenging, such as during illness or major life changes. During these times, it's important to be gentle with oneself and seek support when needed. Remembering that self-care is a fundamental part of maintaining mental and physical health can provide motivation to keep prioritizing it.

Conclusion

Self-care is a vital component of managing postnatal depression and ensuring overall well-being for new mothers. By understanding its importance, implementing practical strategies, and balancing motherhood with self-care, mothers can navigate the challenges of PND more effectively. Real-life examples demonstrate the positive impact of self-care, offering hope and inspiration to others. Moving forward, maintaining self-care practices ensures that mothers can continue to thrive, both for themselves and for their families. Prioritizing self-care is not just an act of self-love; it is an essential step toward a healthier, happier motherhood journey.

11

Preventing Postnatal Depression

Chapter 11: Preventing Postnatal Depression

Postnatal depression (PND) affects approximately one in seven new mothers, making it a significant concern for women navigating the postpartum period. While PND can be a challenging and isolating experience, it is not inevitable. With the right strategies and support, women can take proactive steps to reduce their risk and safeguard their mental health. This chapter delves into the key risk factors associated with PND, explores actionable preventive measures, and underscores the importance of early intervention. By understanding these elements, women can empower themselves to navigate the postpartum period with resilience and confidence.

Understanding the Risk Factors

Postnatal depression is influenced by a combination of biological, psychological, and environmental factors. Hormonal changes, such as the rapid drop in estrogen and progesterone levels after childbirth, play a significant role in mood regulation and can contribute to depressive symptoms. However, hormones are only one piece of the puzzle. A lack of social support, particularly from partners, family, or friends, can leave new mothers feeling isolated and overwhelmed. Previous mental health issues, such as depression or anxiety, also increase the likelihood of developing PND, as does a history of stressful life events, including financial difficulties or relationship challenges.

These factors often interact in complex ways. For example, a woman with a history of depression may find that hormonal changes exacerbate her symptoms, especially if she lacks a support system. Similarly, a mother experiencing financial stress may struggle to prioritize self-care, further increasing her vulnerability to PND. By identifying these risk factors early, women can take targeted steps to mitigate their impact.

Building a Strong Support Network

One of the most effective ways to prevent postnatal depression is to build and maintain a robust support network. This network can include family members, friends, healthcare professionals, and community resources. Emotional support is crucial, as having someone to talk to can alleviate feelings of loneliness and provide a sense of validation. Practical support, such as help with household chores or childcare, can also reduce the physical and mental burden on new mothers.

To build a support network, start by reaching out to trusted individuals before childbirth. Discuss your needs and expectations openly, ensuring they understand how they can assist you during the postpartum period. Joining local or online parenting groups can also provide a sense of community and connection with others who are experiencing similar challenges. Additionally, consider enlisting the help of professionals, such as lactation consultants or postpartum doulas, who can offer specialized guidance and reassurance.

It's important to remember that support is not a one-time offering but an ongoing process. Regularly check in with your network, and don't hesitate to ask for help when needed. Communication is key—expressing your feelings and needs openly can strengthen your relationships and ensure you receive the support you require.

Lifestyle Adjustments for Mental Health

Lifestyle choices play a pivotal role in mental health during the postpartum period. Prioritizing self-care, even in small ways, can make a significant difference. A balanced diet rich in nutrients supports physical recovery and stabilizes mood. Foods high in omega-3 fatty acids, such as salmon and walnuts, are particularly beneficial for brain health. Staying hydrated and avoiding excessive caffeine or sugar can also help regulate energy levels and mood.

Regular exercise, even in gentle forms like walking or yoga, releases endorphins and reduces stress. Physical activity doesn't have to be strenuous; even 10-15 minutes a day can improve mental well-being. Adequate sleep is equally important, though it can be challenging with a newborn. Establishing a sleep routine, such as taking naps when the baby sleeps or sharing nighttime responsibilities with a partner, can help ensure you get enough rest.

Mindfulness and relaxation techniques, such as deep breathing exercises or meditation, can help manage stress and promote emotional balance. These practices encourage you to stay present and cultivate a sense of calm amidst the chaos of new motherhood. Setting aside a few minutes each day for these activities can create a powerful foundation for mental health.

Seeking Professional Guidance Early

Early intervention is critical in preventing postnatal depression from becoming severe or prolonged. If you recognize any risk factors or begin to experience symptoms of PND, seek professional guidance as soon as possible. Healthcare providers, such as obstetricians, midwives, or mental health specialists, can offer valuable support and resources.

Therapy is one of the most effective early intervention strategies. Cognitive-behavioral therapy (CBT) and interpersonal therapy (IPT) are particularly well-suited for addressing the thought patterns and relationship dynamics associated with PND. Therapy provides a safe space to explore your feelings, develop coping strategies, and build resilience.

In some cases, medication may be recommended to manage symptoms of depression. Antidepressants can be a helpful tool, especially when combined with therapy. It's essential to discuss the benefits and risks with your healthcare provider to make an informed decision. Remember, seeking help is a sign of strength, not weakness—early treatment can significantly improve outcomes for both you and your family.

Real-Life Examples and Case Studies

Real-life examples can illustrate the effectiveness of preventive measures and inspire confidence in their application. Consider Sarah, a first-time mother who experienced anxiety during pregnancy. Recognizing her increased risk for PND, she prioritized building a support network by involving her partner and joining a local mothers' group. She also incorporated mindfulness practices into her daily routine, which helped her manage stress and stay grounded. By seeking therapy early and maintaining open communication with her support system, Sarah successfully navigated the postpartum period without developing PND.

Another example is Emily, who struggled with depression in the past. Aware of her vulnerability, she worked with her healthcare provider to develop a preventive plan that included regular exercise, a balanced diet, and ongoing therapy. Emily also enlisted the help of a postpartum doula to assist with childcare, allowing her to focus on self-care. These strategies enabled her to maintain her mental health and enjoy her journey into motherhood.

These stories highlight the importance of proactive measures and demonstrate that prevention is possible with the right tools and support.

Conclusion

Postnatal depression is a common but preventable condition that can significantly impact a mother's well-being and her family's dynamics. By understanding the risk factors, building a strong support network, making lifestyle adjustments, and seeking professional guidance early, women can reduce their vulnerability to PND. Real-life examples underscore the power of these strategies and offer hope to those navigating the postpartum period. Remember, prioritizing your mental health is not just an act of self-care—it's an essential investment in your ability to thrive as a mother and as an individual. With the right knowledge and resources, you can take charge of your postpartum journey and create a foundation of resilience and joy.

12

Moving Forward: Recovery and Hope

Chapter 12: Moving Forward: Recovery and Hope

The journey through postnatal depression (PND) can feel isolating and overwhelming, but it is important to remember that recovery is not only possible—it is within reach. This chapter is designed to provide you with hope, practical guidance, and the tools you need to move forward. By sharing stories of resilience, exploring the long-term outlook for PND, and offering a wealth of resources, we aim to empower you to take control of your mental health and build a brighter future for yourself and your family.

Stories of Recovery: Finding Hope in Shared Experiences

One of the most powerful sources of hope comes from hearing the stories of others who have walked a similar path. Consider Sarah, a mother of two who struggled with PND after the birth of her second child. For months, she felt trapped in a fog of exhaustion, guilt, and sadness. But with the support of her partner, therapy, and a local mothers' group, she gradually regained her sense of self. Today, Sarah not only thrives as a mother but also volunteers as a peer supporter for other women facing PND.

Then there's Priya, who initially resisted seeking help, fearing judgment from her family. When she finally confided in her doctor, she was connected with a therapist specializing in perinatal mental health. Through cognitive behavioral therapy (CBT) and small, daily acts of self-care, Priya learned to challenge negative thought patterns and prioritize her well-being. Her story underscores the importance of reaching out—even when it feels daunting.

These stories, and countless others like them, illustrate a crucial truth: recovery is not linear, and it looks different for everyone. What unites these women is their resilience and their willingness to seek and accept help. If you are struggling, know that you are not alone, and that with time and support, you too can find your way forward.

The Long-Term Outlook: Managing Postnatal Depression

Understanding the long-term trajectory of PND can help you prepare for the road ahead. While many women experience significant improvement within months of beginning treatment, others may find that symptoms linger or resurface during periods of stress. This does not mean you have failed—it simply means you may need to revisit your coping strategies or adjust your support network.

One common misconception is that PND will disappear on its own once the baby grows older. In reality, untreated PND can have lasting effects on both maternal and child well-being. Studies show that children of mothers with unresolved PND may be at higher risk for emotional and behavioral challenges. This is not meant to alarm you, but to emphasize the importance of proactive management.

Preventive measures are key. Regular check-ins with a mental health professional, even after symptoms improve, can help you stay on track. Building a toolkit of coping mechanisms—such as mindfulness exercises, journaling, or physical activity—can also provide a buffer against future stressors. Additionally, open communication with your partner or family about your needs can strengthen your support system and reduce the risk of relapse.

It's also important to address the impact of PND on family dynamics. Partners may feel helpless or overwhelmed, and siblings may sense the tension. Family therapy or couples counseling can be invaluable in fostering understanding and creating a united front in your recovery journey.

Resources for Continued Support: Building a Strong Support System

You do not have to navigate PND alone. A robust support system can make all the difference in your recovery. Below is a curated list of resources to help you access the help you need:

Professional Help

- **Therapists Specializing in Perinatal Mental Health**: Look for clinicians certified by organizations like Postpartum Support International (PSI). Many offer teletherapy, making access easier for new mothers.

- **Psychiatrists**: For those who may benefit from medication, a psychiatrist can provide a tailored treatment plan.

- **Primary Care Providers**: Your GP or OB-GYN can monitor your progress and refer you to specialists as needed.

Community Support

- **Local Support Groups**: Organizations like PSI and The Blue Dot Project host in-person and virtual meetings where you can connect with others who understand your experience.

- **Online Communities**: Forums such as Reddit's r/Postpartum_Depression or private Facebook groups offer anonymity and 24/7 peer support.

Self-Help Tools

- **Books and Workbooks**: *The Postpartum Depression Workbook* by Bethany Warren and *Good Moms Have Scary Thoughts* by Karen Kleiman provide practical exercises and reassurance.
- **Apps**: Mood-tracking apps like Daylio or meditation apps like Headspace can help you stay grounded.

Family and Friends

Educate your loved ones about PND so they can offer meaningful support. Share articles, books, or even this chapter with them to help them understand what you're going through.

Self-Care and Empowerment: Taking Control of Your Mental Health

Self-care is not a luxury—it is a necessity for recovery. Small, consistent actions can have a profound impact on your mental health. Below are practical strategies to incorporate into your daily routine:

Mindfulness and Relaxation
- Start with just five minutes of deep breathing or guided meditation each day.
- Practice grounding techniques, such as naming five things you can see, four you can touch, three you can hear, two you can smell, and one you can taste.

Physical Well-Being
- Gentle exercise, like walking or postnatal yoga, can boost mood and energy levels.
- Prioritize nutrition by preparing simple, nourishing meals. If cooking feels overwhelming, ask a friend or partner to help.

Emotional Boundaries
- Give yourself permission to say no to additional responsibilities. Your primary job right now is healing.

- Delegate tasks when possible, whether it's childcare, household chores, or errands.

Small Wins

Celebrate tiny victories, whether it's taking a shower, reaching out to a friend, or simply getting through a difficult day. Progress is cumulative.

Conclusion: A Future of Hope and Healing

Postnatal depression is a challenging chapter in your life, but it does not define you. By drawing strength from the stories of others, understanding the long-term nature of PND, and leveraging the resources available to you, you can reclaim your sense of self and build a fulfilling life for you and your family.

Recovery is not about perfection—it's about progress. Every step you take, no matter how small, is a testament to your resilience. You are stronger than you know, and with the right tools and support, you will emerge from this experience with newfound wisdom and hope. The road ahead may have its twists and turns, but you are not walking it alone. Together, we can move forward—toward healing, toward joy, and toward a brighter tomorrow.

www.ingramcontent.com/pod-product-compliance
Lightning Source LLC
Chambersburg PA
CBHW071727020426
42333CB00017B/2422